ADVANCE PRAISE

Joe's *Simplify Cancer* podcast is an asset for anyone facing a cancer diagnosis. With this book, he's used his expertise to assemble a valuable guide for dealing with something that many have overlooked in the past—the psychological impact of cancer.

~ Dr. David Palma, MD, PhD, author of *Taking Charge of Cancer*

Hearing the three words "you have cancer" is devastating. Receiving this news is overwhelming. Joe has helped to make the experience a little less stressful by creating simple, easy to understand tools to help those affected by this disease navigate the complexities of Dr. Visits, treatments and so much more.

~ Lee Silverstein, We Have Cancer Podcast Host and Stage IV Survivor

Joe has used his personal experience to craft a simple, practical and meaningful strategy to help others in facing their cancer diagnosis and in taking back some control of their journey. Men facing a new diagnosis are sure to find *Simply Cancer* a great resource.

~ Mike Craycraft R.Ph., Survivor/Founder,
Testicular Cancer Society

Dealing with cancer is tough and can leave people feeling scared and isolated. Joe's been through the wringer and has distilled what he's learnt from his cancer experience into this easily understandable and relatable book, *Simplify Cancer*. He offers personal and practical advice on everything from making an informed treatment decision, to getting support, and managing worries about the future. I hope this book will help those unlucky enough to be affected by cancer feel less alone and that they can live a personally meaningful life wth and beyond cancer.

~ Allan 'Ben' Smith, PhD, Centre for Oncology
Education & Research Translation (CONCERT),
Ingham Institute & UNSW

SIMPLIFY
CANCER

SIMPLIFY
CANCER

Man's guide to navigating
the everyday reality of cancer

Joe Bakhmoutski

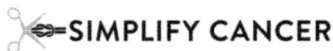

✂=SIMPLIFY CANCER

http://simplifycancer.com

ISBN   978-0-6485995-0-0 (paperback)
          978-0-6485995-1-7 (ebooks)

First Edition

Editor: Daniel Johnson
Cover design: Boris Sabranovic
Interior Design: Adina Cucicov

Disclaimer: This book is not intended as a substitute for the medical advice of physicians.

FOREWORD

THE EXPERIENCE OF CANCER is for most people a major life stress, an experience that brings with it fears about the present and the future, and for many, questions about who we are and what life means. This is perhaps even more so if you are young, have family who depend on you, and if your cancer threatens your sense of self in a personal way. All these things were true for Joe Bakhmoutski when he was diagnosed with testicular cancer. In his book *Simplify Cancer*, Joe shares his personal insights based on his experience and what strategies he developed and employed to effectively manage this challenge. It is a generous step to take and many people will no doubt find a resonance with Joe's experience. Personal experience provides a unique insight from a perspective of having walked this path, and his rich account adds to what we know and can learn.

~ Professor Suzanne Chambers AO

TABLE OF CONTENTS

INTRODUCTION

CANCER IS A BETRAYAL.

Imagine the woman you love, the one woman who shares your deepest secrets, who's there when you're most vulnerable, imagine that your woman is cheating on you.

And as betrayals go, you never see that one coming...

But something tips you off.

Something that wasn't quite right.

Maybe it's one too many late night texts, or another excuse that starts to wear thin.

Maybe it's another story from her past that doesn't add up.

Deep inside, something is wrong and you know it, even when you can't pin it down.

After all, there is no proof. No hard evidence.

What if you're just paranoid, or jealous? Isn't that normal, up to a point?

You cling to even the tiniest glimmer of hope that you got it all wrong, that it's all just one big mistake, that you'd wake up from this nightmare and things would go back to the way they were, the way life ought to be…

Cancer hits you the same way.

If you could only go back to the way it was, the way life was meant to be.

The familiar world where you worry about being late for work.

Where oncologists are locked away in a hospital far, far away.

Where tomorrow is dependable and accounted for.

But…

There's no going back.

The well-trodden, familiar paths for navigating your life have disappeared, once and for all.

I know, because I've been through it all, and I'm here to help.

I'm no medical expert or new age guru, but I lived every word that you read here.

I know what it's like to be scared and numb in the face of a diagnosis.

Screwed over because this was never supposed to happen.

To be angry at your own helplessness, at the mercy of the man in a white coat.

To have everything you know turn upside down, every future shrouded by uncertainty.

To have many of those around you stand idly by because they don't get it—they haven't been through it and don't know how to help.

I will share what worked for me and what I would have done differently, given the choice.

There are no flowery, sugar sweet quotes you can stick on a wall.

This is a 100% honest, unbiased dive into what cancer is really like, including all the everyday things that no one tells you.

I'm going to steer clear of history and medical jargon to focus on practical steps for how you can stop cancer from running your life.

There are four parts to this book, one for each major challenge that cancer forces you to face:

1. Why me?

Like a hit and run, cancer is never expected, fair or just. But you can reign in the onrushing tide of panic and the crushing helplessness of it all. Discover how you can break the chain of non-stop thoughts about cancer.

2. What happens now?

Cancer is so unexpected that you can't help but be unprepared and disoriented. So how do you start dealing with it in a measured, rational way so you can make informed decisions about your treatment? We will cover how to deal with the uncertainty of everyday life, what to expect from treatment, how to work with your medical team, and how to keep your sanity in the midst of it all.

3. Who is going to be there for me through cancer?

It can be awkward talking about cancer, and yet you don't want to sideline people who care about you. We will explore how to rally those people around you without being over-dramatic or dismissive and pushing them away when you need them the most. You can have the support you want, on your terms.

4. How do I deal with uncertainty?

Cancer is like life during wartime, where you are always waiting for something to happen, constantly on guard, expecting bad news. Another treatment, another check-up, the excruciating wait for results... You're always on edge, but there is a way around it. You can put your worries aside to have the life you want despite cancer.

I know this is a tough time right now and I want to make it as easy as possible for you to apply the advice that I share with you...

That's why I created a truly is a one of a kind experience just for you with a truly unique gift bundle to go along with this book.

I am including the Simplify Cancer video course where I walk you through overcoming the four key challenges us men face during cancer, as well as the audiobook version that you can listen to when you're on the go or resting from treatment, and every actionable tool discussed in the book are included free of charge, all in one convenient location!

Here is your super secret URL for you: http://simplifycancer.com/scbookbundle

Thank you for getting this book and dedicating your time and energy to look out for yourself when you are dealing with cancer!

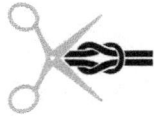

WHY ME?

MY DIAGNOSIS

For weeks, my pants crawl with ants.

It's as if all my underwear has shrunk down three sizes overnight.

I can't sleep, and it's hard to describe this odd feeling that something is off because I can't place it exactly...

So one night in the shower, I reach down to my groin and feel a hard mass.

A cold shudder cuts right through me.

I check again, and the hard lump on my testicle is there, and I can tell it's no good.

It all comes together in an instant.

It's like the Alien movies, when the helpless astronaut can feel a monster in their chest and they know it's about to burst out yet they feel completely powerless to stop it.

The next day, I rush to the doctor's office.

She looks after our entire family, my wife and son; it's hard to talk about something that personal.

I stumble through my symptoms and she listens with intent.

There is a hint of disappointment in her voice as she asks me to have a look at it.

What could be putting her off?

Is it because it's below the belt stuff, and I'm a man?

And then, it dawns on me...

I think, "Wait a second, lady, I know what you might be thinking, but trust me, this is no STD!"

Within seconds, her expression changes and she calls the nearest radiologist.

At the lab, the nurse does my ultrasound.

She rubs oil into my groin and guides the scan arm around it.

Never could I have imagined this moment to be less erotic…

It's so weird, more so because she does it in complete silence and abruptly, then asks me to get dressed and leave.

The atmosphere is uncomfortable. Doesn't she know that I'm not enjoying this either?

Months later I learn that this is because she has found something in the scan but is not allowed to tell me.

Things turn around quickly, and on the same day I find myself in the urologist's office.

There is purpose and innate experience behind the man's expression and practiced movements.

He takes a brief look at the scans.

He leads me to the examination bed and presses around my stomach, then goes carefully over my testicles.

His hands never intrude, despite the fact that he is the first man to ever touch my balls.

I sink into the arm chair and the urologist reveals my fate: "I'm sorry, but this is definitely cancer. We need to operate immediately, I have a time available this Thursday. Can you do it?"

When I get home, tears well up in my eyes.

It's wrong, so wrong, it's never meant to be ME!

What have I done to deserve this?!

Just when everything was going so well...

I can't change it, I can't do a damn thing about it, and I don't even know how deep the rot goes!

What if this is it, that's all there is, the end of the line?

I built my life so carefully, past the betrayals, past my ex, past the struggle of uprooting continents, past those who pointed their fingers, made fun of me, who never believed that I would crawl through life and start winning...

All for nothing!

What will I tell my wife?

My son?

They are going to be home soon, and I need to pull myself together.

Time to speak the words, the words that will get me through this…

You are not alone.

You can do this.

Your best is yet to come.

Yes, even after all this, the best is yet to come.

YOU NEVER SEE IT COMING

Nothing and no one prepares you for cancer.

It explodes into your life with a myriad of epic questions about life, death, and everything in between.

It drives you mad with anger—why me, what have I done to deserve this?

There's a pressing fear—what if the treatment doesn't work?

Is this the end, am I going to die?

Guilt, even—could have I done anything, anything at all to prevent it, or to catch it before it spread?

Anxiety—is the cancer growing?

Could this be happening to me?

When you have cancer shoved in your face, it's difficult to make sense of it—the craziness and the injustice of it all, they get to you. It's so wrong and unfair on every level.

Sometimes you can't stop thinking about it, unspoken fears that are always there, in the back of your mind.

You wrestle with the cancer verdict, numb with the shock of being plunged into the icy depths of the unknown as the reality of cancer refuses to sink in...

Worse than that—the shock of the cancer diagnosis isn't going away.

It prevents you from focusing on your treatment and the life you want despite cancer.

The precise moment of your diagnosis becomes a trap, but it doesn't have to be that way!

You can disconnect yourself from the experience by changing the way you look at it.

Easier said than done, but this is something that changed my entire perspective.

For me, it was a moment where my world crumbled, it lost shape and escaped meaning.

Nothing made sense, and I couldn't change one damn thing...

Time heals all, but this was time I didn't have.

My grandmother told me once: "You have a hard life, without god or ideology to rely on for guidance."

It's true that our ancestors had rituals to acknowledge and process major life events, but what can we do now?

To use the rights of passage within our mind and memory, to go past a trauma that can't be undone, to put it behind you...

This is the time I keep returning to, the moment when I found out I had cancer, I keep replaying it over and over again when I realise that I can't fight nature.

It's resigned to memory, in a place where it can hold me back no more.

I have the power to move forward because I accept the past.

This is the exact process that helped me put the deadweight of the cancer diagnosis behind me to move on with my life.

Try this exercise and see if it fits:

Close your eyes, and sit back.

Imagine you are in a theatre.

There is no one there but you.

You are in your seat, waiting for the show to begin.

You look to the stage, the lights are down, it's very still and quiet...

The curtains crawl off to the side, the lights go up, you look up at the stage, and it's a scene you recognise in an instant...

It's the time you found out you have cancer.

What was that like? Visualise it in front of you.

If you are in your doctor's office, are you sitting down?

What is the first thing that races through your mind?

What are you going to do next?

As your diagnosis unfolds in front of you, you can't help but think that this is something that has already taken place, in the past.

It's in the past, and no matter how crazy your life has been ever since, it's in the past.

You have already lived through it and moved on.

You are not up there in the lights, you are in your seat, and in a way, what's unfolding out there on the stage has nothing to do with you…

Not anymore.

You see it for what it is—a profound shock that has already set in, and now you're dealing with it as best you can.

What you have now is only a memory that holds no sway over you anymore.

So you get up, and you walk away.

You head towards the exit sign that is flashing away in the distance.

You walk away from your diagnosis, away from the shock and the injustice of it all, towards now.

You can't change what happened, but now you are in control of the situation.

Now you can decide where you put your energy and how you're going to take on treatment and the life beyond.

You are done fighting against the sentence that has been handed down to you by fate, and you are taking charge of this new reality of cancer.

Now, open your eyes and take a deep breath.

If this puts some mental or emotional distance between you and your diagnosis, you can play through this scene whenever it gets too much, when you still can't believe you ended up with cancer.

By replaying your diagnosis, it brings you to a place where you can start doing what is within your power to tackle this disease.

This will help you move forward with life and put all your energy into dealing with treatment to have the best life you can despite cancer.

The worst of it is already behind you—the numbing unreality of the diagnosis, the helplessness of it all, the fear of the unknown...

Getting cancer is never deserved, just, or fair, but now, you can start dealing with your disease on your terms.

MOVING FORWARD

You cannot stop cancer from coming into your life, unasked— no one can change that, but we can accept it for what it is.

This is **Accept**, the first step of the three-step process for putting cancer in its place that I call **AIM** because the aim is to set your cancer aside and put it in a place where it's no longer running your life.

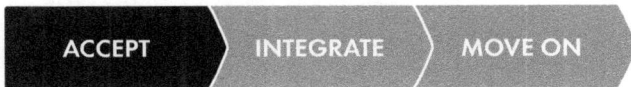

ACCEPT INTEGRATE MOVE ON

Accepting cancer is an opportunity to make peace with it and move forward on your own terms.

Acceptance is not the same as weakness—you are not giving in to fate and circumstance, you are putting a stop to the tyranny of the unknown.

So let's make a deal with cancer, a treaty that spells out how you are going to strip cancer of its power.

This can be your formal agreement with cancer, if you choose. Think of it as your personal mantra, one which you can take around with you wherever you go and repeat as needed, or even write it down and carry it in your pocket:

"You are a part of me,

And it's a part that I don't like.

You appeared out of nowhere, unasked, but I'm willing to live with it…

For now.

You do not, under any circumstances, control my life.

You cannot direct what I do, or don't do.

So let's agree on this…

If you are a part of me, then you will never stop me from living my life the way I want to.

I am going to talk about you with everyone I care about, and I'm going to tell them how I'm doing and how they can be there for me.

I am going to live out my passions and do things I love with people I care about every single day, because with or without you, this is the only life I get.

I am going to find out as much as I can to put you in your place—out of my way.

And when the treatment is done, I want us to go our separate ways.

These are my terms, and this is my last and final offer.

Take it, and leave me be.

Signed,

[Your Name]"

This is a representation of the contract I made with cancer; yours will reflect who you are if you choose to find your own terms.

Make your own version and put it on your wall, or your fridge, next to your bed, anywhere it will serve as a reminder of where you are with it.

Yes, cancer is here, but it's not running your life.

Not anymore. Once you accept this, you can direct your energy and your strength towards treatment and having the life you want despite cancer.

THIS IS NOT THE END

When you find out you have cancer, your life breaks off into two distinct paths.

One road is very much like the life you had before cancer where you get up and spend time on work, your family, and everyday things that need fixing.

The other road is your new reality of living with cancer where you see your oncologist, make decisions about treatment and where you have to consider the possibility that you might actually die.

Right now, these two roads run in opposite directions; they seem to never meet, yet this is an illusion.

You will never go back to the life before cancer.

Because even if things do go to plan, you will never look at your past, your present and your future in the same way again.

You'll make different plans, you'll want to make changes, and that is the natural way forward.

The course has been changed, altered forever.

These two paths need to merge in order to get to the new place without wasting your energy going in the wrong direction.

Your old familiar life has a rhythm and it's filled with things that make you feel normal.

It's a rhythm you are comfortable with…

The alarm signals a new day with the cancer that lives inside you.

You poke around the omelette, gulp down the coffee.

These are the foods that you used to love to kick start the day, but right now, they give you no pleasure, no comfort.

Your wife asks you something about your plans for later.

But your head is elsewhere, and it slips right past.

"What was it you said, honey?"

"I only asked you five minutes ago… Never mind, it's not important."

You suddenly have the thought, "I don't want to die, I don't want to die, I don't want to die…

Get away from me, I want my normal life back!

Give me anything, something to cling to, some shred of certainty, of realness that I can hold in my arms, roll on my tongue, play through my mind.

Just make it through the day, lose myself in the work, anything to chase away these worrisome thoughts."

But they won't go away.

This is when you go to your specialist, you make time for tests, you get treated at the hospital.

You want to keep them separate because you don't want your cancer life to take over... It may be tempting to consider these lives as two roads that should never meet.

But the problem is, you still have your scan results on your mind, and how the treatment is going, and you can't stop thinking about this weird pain that you're having...

It's always in your head and it gets to you that much more, because it's too big and too scary to just stay in the background.

And it's tough because the way things are right now are not what you want them to be...

You want this cancer gone, to never even have happened in the first place, and yet it's here, watching your every move.

You're pulled apart by the constant tension around the way your life is right now versus the way you want it to be, taking away the energy you need for your treatment and your recovery.

The amount of stress and pressure you are under right now is unlike most challenges we have in life.

Right now, you are at the epicentre of a force of nature that demands a response and you can't afford wasting energy.

There is so much going on and you are bound to spread yourself thin when you do more than you can take on.

This is when you start overthinking everything and getting down on yourself.

For me, I began catching myself in the act of telling people what they want to hear and realised how pointless that was.

"Who am I kidding?

This is cancer, it's supposed to be hard!"

So I became more honest and direct about my life, about things that were hard to talk about, things that put me on edge.

When my wife asked me how my day was, I told her about my worries around returning to work after treatment.

I told her about the support I had from folks on the testicular cancer forum and how that made me more prepared.

It helped me to open up about things that were bothering me and it made things easier for her to relate to my struggle.

When my boss asked me about how I'm getting on, I said I'm worried about how long it will put me out of action for.

He was adamant that I needed to look after myself first and made sure I knew that the job would still be there when I'm ready.

That made things easier as I didn't have to worry about work during treatment.

When my friend asked me how my day was, I told him I'm freaking out about starting chemo and staying at the hospital.

He came to visit me at the hospital and brought me a new book, which cheered me up and made it easier to pass the time.

When you make cancer a part of your everyday life, you don't need to find the right thing to say or always be the hero. By opening up about what you are going through, you are having a real conversation about things that matter, with genuine people who care!

And it's hard to find the right time, or the words to talk about it with people in your life.

You don't want them to feel sorry for you, or to look like you can't handle it.

Or worse, you don't want to add to their troubles and be a burden.

But this way, you're not making things easier for anyone—at least not for anyone who cares about you!

Because the most important thing for this person is to know what's happening in your world, what you are worried about, and how they can help, even if only by being around you.

There's nothing worse then second guessing someone you love.

This is the **Integrate** part of our **AIM** framework, where you make cancer a part of your life in order to become more connected to your values and your people.

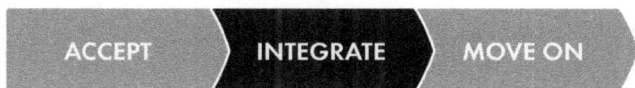

ACCEPT   INTEGRATE   MOVE ON

These two lives, one without cancer, and one where you force your way through treatment, they are one and the same.

Like siblings, they need to coexist without too much conflict, they need to live beside each other because that is the best way forward.

There is no need to resist what has already taken place.

We accept the challenge, we meet it with honour and look towards the future.

The best way to fuse these two lives together is through open communication with your people.

How do you know what the person next to you is thinking about right now?

You don't—unless they tell you about it!

It's no good guessing—even when you know the person well, you could still be off track.

We expect support and understanding from people around us, but it can be hard to relate when you haven't lived through the experience.

And they don't want to say the wrong thing or do the wrong thing to make you feel sorry for yourself or as if you can't handle trouble on your own.

It's true that family, friends and people you work with, they want to be there for you in a meaningful way, but they don't know how.

So we need to guide them, to show them how to support you in a way that helps you and your life right now.

Let them know:

- What's on your mind?
- What's bothering you right now?
- What's keeping you up at night?
- What scares you the most, and why?
- What do you need?
- What would make your life easier?

If you have a partner, you can use the times you spend together on a regular basis to have a conversation.

Even if for only five minutes a day—do whatever you need to keep your partner from guessing about where you're at.

Don't keep your family, friends and coworkers guessing on what is the right thing to say or do...

Tell them—be as explicit as you can be!

It's easy to send a group email—this way, you don't have to repeat yourself every time!

Get your close friends or family to come with you to your specialist appointment to keep you company so that they know exactly what you're going through.

People who truly care about you are going to be grateful because you just made it easy for them to support you!

This is what **Integrate**, the second part of our **AIM** conversation, is all about—charting the course away from uncertainty to lead the life you want despite cancer.

HOW TO LIMIT YOUR WORRIES

It only takes one worrisome thought to trigger a chain reaction of more worries, and before you know it, they start to multiply and grow, one after another, day after day.

What started with a random headache now has you thinking about much weightier things, like dying miserable and alone.

And then, you forget that it was a fairly innocent symptom that got you roped into these depressing thoughts in the first place.

You're on edge, you are freaking out, and you don't even know why!

You want to get rid of those worries when they first come up.

You want to draw those worries out in the open, break them apart, examine each one, and find the best way to deal with it.

It's like an argument with your partner that got you angry over a minor comment, a misunderstanding that leads down the path of remembering all the nasty things this person has said or done in the past.

Petty, insignificant arguments can snowball into awkward, misshapen issues that hang over you.

They can destroy your mood unless you dig deep and find out the root cause of the problem.

Once you understand what that is, you can examine it closer and decide what to do about it.

These are the difficult conversations that you've got to have...

There is no way around it—bring whatever is bothering you into the open so that you can deal with it and get on with your life.

A powerful way to get these worries out is to write them down on paper.

When you have a list of worries in front of you, you are already hot on the trail of what's really bothering you the most and how it got to you in the first place. You will also breathe easier when you get things off your chest.

It's for your eyes only so there is no need to filter anything out or find the right words to tell your worry the right way. And some worries are bound to surprise you.

When you turn off your filters, there will be things you never even considered because they are hiding deep in your head.

You can find a solution that did not come to mind before because you never had the chance to look at the bigger picture and assess the situation in its entirety.

When it's written down in front of you, your thoughts become points on a map.

You instantly understand how things stand, where you're at and which direction you should head into now. Like the man who's wife is cheating on him—you're often the last one to find out.

He is so caught up in the situation that he can't tell the obvious, but everyone around him can tell she's flirting with another man and has zero interest in her husband.

Zooming out of the immediate situation brings clarity—you pinpoint the problem and decide what to do next! As you practice getting your thoughts out and letting yourself see them, your worries are going to become more manageable.

Right now, these things that are bothering you, they build on top of one another, they blend together and you can't even tell them apart!

So you have this giant storm cloud of uncertainty hanging over you, and it's not getting any smaller...

But when you extricate your worries out of your mind and onto the paper, there is no room to hide from them anymore...

It's out of your head, out in the open; you can see each worry for what it is and find a way around it.

Use this prompt to get your worries to come out of hiding:

> *"The thing that scares me the most about cancer right now is..."*

And start writing!

Don't think about it—just go for it.

I prefer pen and paper to write on, but use whatever works for you—your phone, your computer, or a voice recorder.

Now that you have a list of worries, examine each one and challenge it:

- Why does it bother me?
- What's behind it? Is there another reason than the obvious?
- Who can help me with that?
- What is the next step I can take to resolve it? Analyse your fears and work out a plan of action immediately.

Let me share two quick examples from my own experience:

> *"What scares me the most about cancer right now is that I won't be able to work, I will lose my job, and we'll have no money to live on."*

I never admitted this to myself in those terms before and after writing it down I realised that I needed to do something about it.

So I explained to my manager that my treatment was going to play out in the next three months and when I am expecting to return.

He reassured me that life comes first and set things in motion to redistribute my workload for the next three months.

His support gave me the much needed peace of mind when it comes to money.

Another worry:

> *"What scares me the most about cancer right now is that the treatment won't work and I'm going to die."*

I could not wait for things to take their turn when confronted with the harsh reality of dealing with cancer… So to sort out this worry, I got the opinion of my specialist as the medical expert and cancer survivors on the online forums who went through this experience and were able to relate.

My oncologist reassured me about my chances and explained what we can do if things didn't go according to plan.

I also reached out to people on the testicular cancer forum with questions and their encouragement and support was immense.

This is **Move On**, step three of our **AIM** path towards peace of mind during cancer, to move on with your life despite worries and uncertainty.

No more nasty surprises—you know what's coming your way and how to deal with it.

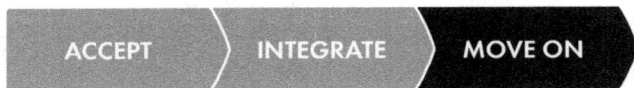

ACCEPT ⟩ INTEGRATE ⟩ MOVE ON

To save yourself the trouble of repeating the same things over and over again, choose your preferred method of sharing your experience with people you care about.

You can talk about your wild ride through cancer in a blog, video, or email, or share your experience on social media— even something as simple as posting a story about treatment, where the hospital is located, or news of a scan result.

You decide how to tell the story, how much you want to share, and who to include in on it.

Another way to move on from your worries is to set some time aside each day to worry about cancer.

When a worrisome thought pops into my head, I can say to myself—I'm going to worry about it later.

Once you have set worry time aside (I suggest 10 minutes), you can then go on with your day, and when that time comes, you circle back to it.

Give yourself the space and time to think about each worry and figure out whether there is anything you can do about it.

If there is, what would be the first step that you can take to solving it?

Set aside five minutes of worry time before dinner, or 10 minutes when you can go for a walk.

You choose what works well for you, but just don't use your worry time before you go to bed or you'll run the risk of snowballing thoughts keeping you up all night.

When you have a process for dealing with worry, you start doing it on autopilot!

This will channel your energy away from tension and into action, into a flow where you are in control of your thoughts, plans, and decisions.

STOP CANCER FROM RUNNING YOUR LIFE
Some say: "I won't let cancer define me."

But how can it not?

It affects what you do every single day, how you think about the future, and the way you see yourself.

So it is with every major life change—whether you change careers, lose a friend or fall in love—you must continuously adapt to what is happening around you.

This personal evolution is what makes you who you are and it's this very same reason why you are not the same person you were before cancer.

So, for better or worse, cancer changes you, but you have the power to choose how it will define you! This brings me back to a moment that nearly cost me my life, and the harsh lesson I learned that day coming face to face with a powerful force of nature.

This story takes place before cancer, on a deserted ocean beach at the end of the world.

It's a perfect day on the ocean—there's an endless horizon of water, a carefree atmosphere.

I am basking in the afternoon glow with soothing sounds of the ocean around me.

I'm swaying back and forth with the waves, obeying their gentle rhythm.

But then, things start to change…

It's a subtle shift I can't quite place, but that I know is wrong.

I try to stand, but my feet can no longer find the ocean floor.

I catch a glimpse of the shoreline and head towards it.

It's so close, I should be out on the sand in no time at all, but my stroke is not getting me anywhere.

I'm stuck, rooted to the spot. I double the effort, but it's no use!

This force is holding me back, an invisible barrier between me and shore.

The waves grow bigger all around me and one hits me square in the face.

I can taste the salty brine in my mouth, and that's when panic set in...

Arms flailing, I call out:

Help! Help! Somebody help me!

In that instant, a man appears amidst the waves and word-lessly helps me onto a surfboard, guiding us towards land.

He helps me onto the sand, and I gasp for air, shocked.

"The rip got you," he says.

"It's a powerful underwater current that you can't fight, you don't want to swim against the rip because it will always pull you in!

Go with it sideways—this is your best way to safety."

And so it is with cancer—the constant worry and uncertainty, the injustice of it all, they are inevitable…

But what if you don't fight against it? What if you could channel your energy in a different direction?

When you go along with the current, when you take cancer on as a set of distinct problems that have solutions, you put yourself in control of the situation.

You decide:

Are you going to drown yourself in pity and misery, or look for ways to get around the inevitable worry and pain that comes with cancer?

Are you going to take things as they come, or take charge of your future and make informed decisions about treatment and recovery?

Will you suffer alone, or speak up about your struggle so you can get the support you want, on your terms?

Will you beat yourself up about the mistakes you made and roads not taken, or create a legacy that serves the people you care about?

Are you going to stay chained to the commitments you never asked for in the first place, or do more of the things you love?

Are you going to dwell on the past, or live in the now, giving in to the moment wholly and without reservations?

Now is the only time you ever get, it's raw and immediate.

It gives you the strength to go on, because real power comes from making peace with uncertainty.

Nothing can stand between you and your way of life—not cancer, not the fear of death.

You walk on through with your head held high, with the dignity that befits you now, a life you worked hard to earn.

You've evolved far beyond the outdated clichés about masculinity, or dominating others.

Your strength comes from connecting the reality inside you to the world beyond your self.

First, when you are connected to your inner circle (your family and friends), you have the support you need to get through treatment and have the life you want beyond cancer.

What's more, you take personal charge in ensuring that your friends and family have the relative peace of mind they need when they understand your worries and how you work through them.

Nothing is worse than being excluded and in the dark about things that matter to you, right?

Second, when you are connected to your outer circle (your medical team and cancer survivors), you can be confident knowing what to expect every step of the way.

When you know how things are likely to turn out, you can put a plan in place to deal with those likely outcomes.

Third, when you are connected to your values and beliefs, you can take a stand on things that are meaningful to you and your life.

This is what gives you the strength to go on and deal with the inevitable curveballs you get from dealing with cancer.

WRAP-UP AND ACTION STEPS

You are in charge of your life during cancer when you are:

✔ Prepared for dealing with the inevitable worry and uncertainty

---

✔ Informed about treatment, including side effects, symptoms, milestones

---

✔ Connected to your friends, family and your medical team

So much of your energy goes into accommodating uncertainty and the stress of dealing with the unknown, but you can channel your energy in a different direction, away from worry and into action when you start to believe that you can get through cancer on your terms!

Yes, cancer has gate-crashed your life, and yes, you've got to plan around it, it's the truth you accept now.

There is no way back now, only forward!

Let's take a long, hard look at each of the beliefs below and see if they sync up with your own:

✔ I believe that cancer is never just or fair and it makes no sense at all.

✔ I understand that none of this is my fault.

✔ I accept that for the time being, cancer is part of my life and I will plan my life around it as best I can.

_____

_____

_____

_____

✔ I am going to be informed about treatment options so that I can make the best decisions for me moving forward.

_____

_____

_____

_____

_____

✔ I am going to be prepared for treatment so that I know what to expect.

_____

_____

_____

_____

_____

✔ I will use every tool at my disposal to deal with stress and worry during cancer.

✔ I will be connected with people I care about by being direct and honest about how they can help me get through this.

You, my friend, did not choose cancer.

It exploded into the familiar, measured life you own, but it doesn't own you.

In fact, you don't owe cancer one damn thing.

Or anyone, for that matter!

And you have no need for sympathy, or worse, pity.

You are here, at the pointy end of bad luck, but you are not alone!

You are one of us, one of many souls trying to stay afloat in the sea of uncertainty,

We are here, and we want to help!

Next, we'll talk about some practical ways to deal with treatment.

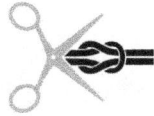

WHAT HAPPENS NOW?

HOW TO MINIMISE STRESS DURING TREATMENT

No one hands you a guide book on the mind games that come along with cancer.

There may be a wealth of information on procedures and physical health considerations, but what about the mental toll? Your life is now a maze of medical tests, specialist appointments, and treatment choices that you have to navigate and work around.

The routine checks for tumor markers, reminders of survival rates, and trips to oncology wards change your way of life. Reality itself becomes alien, and yet, you remain the person you have always been—a man who stands by his decisions and his core values.

When you hit a wall, you don't give up—you pick yourself up and find ways around it, adapting to your ever-changing environment.

This adaptability is the one thing that cancer will never take from you, and it is what will ultimately allow you to stay true to who you are so you can have the best life you can in spite of your disease.

This is something that never changes; you can always stay true to who you are and deal with challenges in the best way you can.

But that's tough when you get cancer because from now on, you expect things to go wrong.

Your experience is now driven by strong emotions, by worry and fear. So how do you keep these powerful undercurrents from impeding your natural resourcefulness? The key is to shift away from emotions towards logic so that you can see things as they are.

One way to do this is to try stepping back from the situation and think of the bigger picture. Here are seven reasons why you should have high hopes for making it through:

1. There is no better time in history to go through this. Doctors and scientists are getting better at discovering

new ways around cancer every day, and there are better ways of dealing with cancer than ever before.

2. Your specialist is not making arbitrary decisions based on a hunch; your treatment is proven to work, and your doctor's advice and treatment plans are driven by evidence-based research, not subjective opinions.

3. Treatment guidelines for most situations rely on the best practice from top experts worldwide.

In most cases, your specialist should be able to explain to you the rationale behind why they are recommending a certain treatment.

If you are not clear about the reasons or not comfortable with the proposed way forward for any reason, ask your doctor for a referral to get a second opinion with another specialist.

Some good questions to ask include: Is this treatment following international guidelines? Have you reached out to an expert in this particular type of cancer? Have you presented my case to a tumor board in your hospital?

You can also reach out by email to experts who specialise in treating a specific type of cancer.

4. Gone are the days where your doctor talks down to you. There was a time when doctors did not listen to patients out of a sense that they knew your situation better than you.

But today, you are not only a part of the conversation, you are the one who makes treatment choices.

And it makes sense—after all, no one knows what's right for you and your life like you know yourself.

But be wary if you get an old school, take it or leave it doctor.

If you're in the dark about what's going on, or you're on edge every minute of the day, you don't need to put up with it any longer.

Don't let anyone sideline you from your treatment, find someone who will listen!

If you're not happy with your specialist for any reason, ask for a referral to someone who gets you and where you're coming from.

Your medical team is there to answer your questions so that you are in control of your life with cancer, not bring more stress into your life.

5. There are options outside of standard treatments.
   A clinical trial is often the best way to get access to the latest treatment available for your cancer.

   Ask your specialist if there any the clinical trials that you can join—these will give you more treatment options to consider.

6. Practitioners with expertise around cancer have re-designed proven therapies to help you get back on track after treatment.
   From exercise and nutrition to mindfulness and yoga, there are many ways to help you heal faster mentally and physically. Every major city will have options to choose from, and there are plenty of resources online and in books to explore.

7. In most cases, there are additional treatment options when things don't go to plan.
   Often times the worst thing about your treatment is not knowing if it's going to work.

You always want to be clear that there is a backup plan just in case.

Don't guess, be explicit and ask your specialist:

- How do we know if this treatment is working and when?
- What happens if this treatment doesn't work as expected?
- What else can we try?

This will give you a relative peace of mind that your treatment has been carefully orchestrated to focus on what's right for you and your life!

When you expect the best from your treatment and your medical team, you know what's coming your way and how to deal with it.

The trouble with expectations is they are usually about things you can't control.

Expectations are how we want the outside world to be, but what about your own thoughts and feelings? How do you expect to be on the inside?

These are what I call inspectations—how you see yourself now that cancer is here.

It's important to always check with what you expect from your internal processes and develop an ongoing relationship with how you're dealing with things.

No matter what the media says, having cancer does not make you a hero.

None of us are—you are just a real man who is going through a tough time, trying to get through this as best as you can.

Chances are, a major part of your identity has been about putting energy into helping your partner, your family, and your friends. You might even be the sole provider or a source of motivation to people in your life.

And that is a great way to be, but things are different now that you are going through cancer.

Now is the time to put yourself first, for your sake and for the sake of those you care about the most.

There are many things you because they need to be done.

We put fun things off for later, but there isn't always a later.

If you have time, what would you do for you and nobody else?

I'm not talking about things that you do out of habit, or out of necessity.

What do you look forward to?

What do you get so immersed in that you lose track of time?

What is something you'd do so much more of if given the chance?

Or is there something you love doing, something you lose yourself in, but life has always gotten in the way?

When you shift your priorities, your life becomes aligned to get you through treatment with the least amount of stress possible.

So, are you doing at least one thing that you love, every single day?

When you do more of what you want, you reduce the amount of stress you are under, and that is what counts the most when you're going through cancer treatment.

Well, with cancer, you have definitive proof that you can't put anything off until later, so the best time to start is now!

Sure enough, there will always be things you can't avoid or people who drag you down, but what can you do now to minimise the number of stressful situations you find yourself in?

Having less stress to carry will give you more energy so you can physically take on more during treatment.

Less worry means you have more headspace to think through things yourself, without distractions, so you can focus on your medical team and being around your family and friends.

When you are not distracted, you are truly there, present, in the moment.

You're listening, responding, asking questions, and having conversations about things that actually matter.

So what can you put off to the side, even if only for a while?

If work is stressing you out, can you work from home on a regular basis, switch to part-time, or redistribute some of your workload?

If there is tension with someone in your life who you can't avoid, can you think of a way to spend time with them in a way that is less painful?

Finding neutral ground when you go out somewhere or spending time in a group is great for breaking old patterns and routines.

I'm now at a place in my life where I have a hard time convincing myself to spend time with people I "should" make time for.

It's not even a choice—I don't have the mental space for it anymore!

Of course, you should still make room for things that need to be done, but there is no reason to do things when your heart is not in it. This will only exacerbate your stress and might create more of a rift between you and these people.

When you are done with treatment, you can once again devote yourself to those people in your life that you can't be without, but now is your time to put yourself first so that you are in the best shape possible for life beyond cancer!

When you put yourself first, you can focus on what's coming your way and how to deal with it.

When you are prepared, the unknown becomes familiar.

The overwhelming turns manageable.

The uncertain is now expected.

The daunting becomes assured. Let's be honest—you are not going to enjoy this whole cancer thing, but having less stress will create the right environment for your cancer treatment.

For me, it became an absolute necessity.

A difficult conversation with my manager meant I did not have to worry about returning to work.

Saying no to an invitation that I wasn't actually interested in made it easy to spend my time doing things I cared about.

It gave me the space to be on my own to go for a walk or a drive to clear my head.

I did not have to worry about commitments and phone calls, I had my own space where I didn't have to listen or respond, I was alone with myself, enjoying the silence.

When you eliminate your worries one at a time, your mind becomes more clear and you are totally focused on what your specialist has to say about treating your cancer.

HOW TO FIND THE RIGHT SPECIALIST

Your first specialist visit hammers home the reality of cancer—yes, this IS happening, and it's happening to you, of all people!

And now you're living your life in the waiting room, never knowing what will come next…

Now is the time when you have trust in the process and trust in the advice that you're getting from your medical team.

So when you are heading for treatment, it is crucial to work with someone who is right for you.

When your specialist understands your concerns, then the treatment is not based on what they know, but what's right for you and your life.

You want the person who's got your back and your best interests at heart, a confidante—that is the difference between therapy and true healing.

I have met with many people in the oncology space, both through treatment and the Simplify Cancer podcast, and these folks are incredible!

It takes a lot of guts and dedication to do what they do and they are on your side, helping you through treatment.

You can be sure that they will be there for you, you can trust their advice, and have confidence that they will look after you.

Your specialist is more than just a doctor whose job it is to work with the disease—they're your champion and trusted advisor who is going to guide you through the dark woods of cancer.

That's why it's important to make a conscious decision to trust that person, completely and without reservations…

Be explicit and write it out with a pen and paper so you can internalise this belief for yourself:

> *"I trust my specialist and my medical team to do the right thing by me and I can talk to them about any concern or worry I have."*

And if you are not on the same wavelength for whatever reason, then it's time for a change.

Don't wait—find the right person to look after you!

When faced with a choice of either chemotherapy or radiation for treating my cancer, I had a tough decision to make.

There were pros and cons for each option: while radiation was less intrusive and had fewer side effects, it could cause another cancer later on in life.

I hoped that a radiation oncologist would help me make a decision.

The radiologist's office was like the inside of a wardrobe—warm to the point of suffocating.

"I understand you are looking at treatment options."

"I am."

The man stared at some incalculable point, far beyond the wall.

"With this cancer, your chances of survival are considerably high with either radiation therapy or chemotherapy."

Oh, that's comforting, I thought. But there was one thing I needed to know...

"Doctor, what are my chances of getting another cancer as a result of this?"

"Well, it's hard to say with all the changes we've had and our new equipment, and in any case, you won't have to worry about it for at least another 10 years".

"Look, in 10 years my son will be starting secondary school, so I'm hoping to stick around for a while. What are the chances of a nasty cancer, if you were to ballpark it?"

His eyebrows jumped and he fidgeted about in his seat as if it was an exam.

"That depends on the radiology equipment. The technology, and how we calibrate it, has moved in leaps and bounds, and we don't have a good point of reference"

I couldn't take it anymore.

"Look, I just want a simple answer! Can you give me a number I can understand?"

And that's what ultimately decided my course of treatment—my trust in the person in front of me.

I went with the oncologist who gave me the chemotherapy and I never looked back.

Trust is always a choice, a hard choice, but one that needs to be there so you can release your worries from the inside of your mental cage into the open field where your specialist, doctor, or nurse can tackle it.

Out there, your worries have nowhere to hide and they are no longer able to spin plots against you.

If your guide is not right for you, you owe it to yourself and those you care about to act quickly to get a second opinion as soon as you can.

There are three ways you can find a different specialist that will guide you through cancer:

- Ask your primary doctor for advice (in person)
- Seek out advice on specialists in your area from a cancer forum (online)
- Contact your local cancer non-profit (phone)

You could start the conversation with something like this:

"Hi my name is _____, *here is my situation... This person is not right for me. Who can you recommend instead, and why?"*

It's as simple as that—the only reason you need to change your specialist is that something doesn't feel right.

This is not an indictment on them as medical expert—doctors understand that like any people who interact with one another, there are different personalities at play and there are times when you don't click with someone.

And that's perfectly fine!

It's just like someone's taste in music—the song that has me weeping with joy might make you puke your guts out!

You are right for acting in your own best interests—don't wait, don't hesitate, and act quickly when it's not working out the way it should.

Trust your gut on this!

This is a critical time in your life and you can't afford to leave things to chance.

PREPARE FOR THE FIRST SPECIALIST VISIT

While your specialist is there to guide you through treatment, you still want to be prepared to address things that are bothering you the most right now.

When you get your questions answered, you will know what to expect and how to deal with what's coming your way.

Sorting through things you want to ask can make a huge difference for your peace of mind down the track!

When it comes to cancer, worries are inevitable, and they will eat away at you every day unless you sort them out.

The only way to do this is to get guidance from your medical team—your specialist, your oncology nurses, and your doctor.

This was what I went through when I found out about the potential of a nasty side effect from Bleomycin, one of the drugs in my chemotherapy cocktail.

It turned out that this drug can cause permanent lung damage severe enough that it requires you to be hooked up to a machine for the rest of your life, or even worse, kills you.

Sure, the chances are less than five percent, which is low enough, but the odds of me getting testicular cancer in the first place were even lower…

"So what's stopping that from happening to me now?!" I thought.

"If I'm stuck to a machine, I'm a living corpse, not a man!

I can't do things around the house, can't go to the beach with my wife, I can't play with my son…

This is no life at all, I'd be better off dying!"

I couldn't stop thinking about it, until I decided to talk it out with my specialist.

He told me that before each round of chemo, we would do a lung function test to verify that my lungs were coping.

We would check in with my breathing throughout the treatment and this chemotherapy regime would change if my lung damage began to rise.

It made things so much easier—I knew there was a plan in place to monitor what was going on and that we could pivot if needed.

But you will only find out about it if you speak up about your worries!

So give yourself five to 10 minutes to stop and think about what you need to figure out.

Write down a list of the things that bother you the most when it comes to treatment and life beyond cancer.

What keeps you up at night?

What is bothering you right now?

What are you worried about when you think about the future?

Use your phone or a pen and paper to take notes when you go to see your specialist.

Here are some of the questions you can ask your specialist:

What are my treatment options?

Which is the best way to go and why?

Can you tell me what it's like?

Will I still be able to do X?

What can I do about Y side effect if it comes up?

What happens if I don't go through with this type of treatment?

When will the treatment/operation take place and how can I prepare?

You may think you know what you are going to ask, but there's a lot going on and it's so easy to forget something or leave out some crucial detail that might be incredibly important to you later on.

Trust me, you won't regret bringing a list of questions!

To save yourself some time, go ahead and grab my free one-page First Oncologist Visit Checklist to take with you: http:// simplifycancer.com/1st-oncologist-visit/

This is a simple PDF with key questions to get you started— just print it, fill it out and take it with you!

There is enough space next to each question for you to make notes during your visit.

And while writing things down is great, it also helps to have an audio recording as backup too.

You can listen to it at any time to clear up any confusion or things you forgot, and you don't need any extra tools or equipment, just your phone.

Do a trial run beforehand to make sure you don't run out of storage space and that the microphone works as it should.

Most specialists will be more than happy for you to record the conversation, but do ask them at the start:

"Is it okay if I record our conversation? I just want to make sure I won't miss anything."

Now that you plan to record the conversation with your specialist, replay key points to ensure you are on the same page, and make brief notes along the way, there is only thing left to do—bring someone along to be a second pair of eyes and ears.

This will ensure that you don't miss out on a crucial point during your visit.

And that's easy to do—there is so much going on that it's easy to forget something important, or miss it altogether!

After every visit, I would check in with my wife: "Was it the following Monday I go back for the follow up infusion? Did he say we have to do day oncology first or head straight to the ward?

Plus it's important to have someone help you take your mind off things, because time stretches out to infinity when you're on the way to the hospital...

And it gets worse in the waiting room—it's like waiting for the execution!

So it helps to bring your partner, or a friend—someone who is going to keep you company and distract you from worry.

They can help you take your mind off things and talk about something other than cancer.

You're about to find out something that could change your life in a big way, and it's good to have someone you trust there to share it with!

It's important to set the expectations with your friend from the start:

> *"I'd love for you to be there with me and just listen so we can compare notes later."*

Chances are, you are going to have questions after the appointment, so it also helps to set up a follow up appointment to clear things up.

Being prepared puts you on the path to staying sane through treatment and keeping it together, for your sake and for those who matter in your life.

HOW TO MAKE THE RIGHT DECISION ABOUT TREATMENT

When it comes to cancer treatment, you expect your specialist to tell you what to do, but often, that's not actually how things work.

You might have different treatment options, each with their pros and cons—so how do you make the right choice?

It's tough because you are now facing life and death decisions over things you don't even fully understand, but it's also an opportunity to take back control of your life during cancer.

Let's be honest, when you find out you have cancer, you become a slave to the medical system.

All of a sudden, random people are telling you what to do:

"Here, fill out another useless form."

"Make an appointment at the most inconvenient time because it's the only one available."

"I don't want you to worry, but here is a long list of nasty side effects that can ruin your life."

Your entire existence now revolves around someone else's schedule, and you lose so much control over what's going on around you that your decision over treatment becomes a real opportunity to wrestle your power back from cancer.

Yes, it's scary and you have no guarantees about the choice you make, and yet...

The balance has changed.

You are in charge now!

You are the one making decisions about your future, and that's how you are going to wrestle your power back from cancer! When you start making informed decisions about what's right for you and your life, you **Accept** that you are going to be prepared for what's coming your way and how to deal with it.

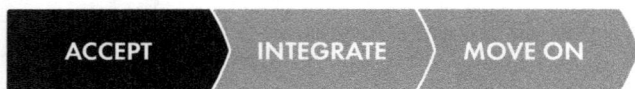

Being prepared means that you:

- Make informed decisions about treatment
- Know how to deal with side effects when they come up
- Get the support you want from people in your life when you need it
- Know when to raise a red flag with your specialist or nurse
- Can manage your energy so that you are not wearing yourself down

- Have a plan for what to do when things don't go to plan
- Focus on having the life you want beyond cancer

This way, you become an expert on your own illness and you know exactly what to expect from treatment every step of the way.

The boundaries of the unknown melt away and you can deal with whatever is thrown at you.

But how do you go about ensuring that you will choose the direction that's right for you right now?

From the very start, you want to go beyond the superficial information you got in the standard handout from the hospital.

These are often filled with meaningless bullet points and generic statements and only serve to confuse you more.

To make a decision that is right for you and your life from this point on, we need to dig deeper.

You want to know exactly how these treatments work and how they would affect you.

Ask your specialist targeted, specific questions about the pros and cons of each treatment option so that you can decide what's right for you and your life.

Here are some examples of questions to ask:

Does this type of treatment provide better chances of curing cancer?

What are the chances of complications?

What side effects do I need to worry about?

How long does it take to recover?

Does it affect my sex life?

Will I be able to have children?

How will it impact my ability to work?

How will it impact my day to day?

How will you know the treatment is working and when?

What are your options if things don't go to plan?

What are the side effects? Can you plan for them in advance (fertility, for example)? And which ones in particular do you need to watch out for (such as lung function or fever spike)?

Let's start with a fact finding mission:

Spend 10 to 15 minutes reading at least three to five articles about your treatment on a reputable, evidence-based website.

These include large not-for-profits such as Cancer Council in Australia, National Cancer Institute in the United States, or MacMillan Cancer Support in the United Kingdom.

Evidence-based research relies on the scientific method—this is your safeguard against speculation and false hope.

Look for clues that apply to you and then figure out the realistic chances for your specific stage/type/situation.

Now that you have a good grasp on how your treatment will play out, you are going to have more questions about it!

We all do—and while your specialist is there to guide you, there is nothing like hearing about it from people who went down that road before.

They've already been at the crossroads where they had to make the same decision that you need to make right now.

And more than anything—they want to help you, because they know exactly what it's like to be scared, lost, and confused.

You can find this kind of guidance in person through a face to face support group, but the easiest way is to find groups online where you can reach out to people who have been through it before.

When you find an online forum for your type of cancer, you can post a question you have about treatment, side effects, or anything else that you're unsure about.

The other nice thing about these communities are that discussion forums leave each topic like a trail so that you can see the kinds of answers people have given to questions, so even if you are not yet ready to reach out to people, you can still benefit from their advice.

When you make a post, the title is like an email's subject line and can tell the reader if this is a conversation where they can contribute.

Like a headline, it's going to need to stick out to the person who you're trying to get to read it!

The body of the topic is where you describe where you're at, what's bothering you and what you want to find out.

Check out my free Online Community Guide with the top three communities listed for your type of cancer on http://SimplifyCancer.com under the Tools section.

More likely than not, people are going to respond to your question in a matter of hours, which gives you almost instant feedback.

And even though every person's experience is somewhat different, you will be able to pick out enough advice to gauge how it applies to you.

There's no limit to how much you can take advantage of the resources available to you. Experiment with your own questions and forums until you feel like you've educated yourself to the degree you need to keep going with confidence.

PREPARED FOR TREATMENT
Often in life, we are forced to rush into a new challenge unprepared.

So it is with cancer—you plunge into it headfirst, forced to figure out new rules, roles, and vocabulary.

It's kind of like school, where learning new things is not the responsibility of the teacher—they may be doing their best to convey the information in an engaging way, but the rest is up to you.

You know what you want and that is what drives you onward.

After all, no one cares about you more than you do!

You know what's right for you and your life, and you don't want to delegate this responsibility to anybody else. Similarly, there are limitations to the way the medical system is set up to work.

Your experience with cancer is a series of events involving different people along the way—the general practitioner who refers you to a specialist, radiologists who will administer your medical scans, nurses who take blood samples and administer treatment, specialists who direct your treatment, surgeons who can remove the tumors…

Every interaction is based on a specific goal and no one is looking at the big picture…

No one, but you!

It's up to you to take charge of the situation and orchestrate the entire experience in a way that makes sense for you and your life, and in order to take control of the situation, you need to understand your disease and everything surrounding it.

When you understand your disease, you disarm cancer's most potent weapon—uncertainty.

You take your power back when you know how things can turn out and what you can do about them.

Do your own research through reputable websites, books, online forums for your type of cancer—any way you can to be in control of the situation.

You can even get the facts straight from the source by reading through articles on a reputable, evidence-based website.

Most countries have large not-for-profit organisations that provide cancer support services. These organisations help people find their way around cancer, and they strive the make their website readable and easy to navigate.

These include:

- Cancer Council (Australia)
- National Cancer Institute (United States)
- Macmillan Cancer Support (United Kingdom)

When you go to an organisation's website, search for your type of treatment and spend at least 10 to 15 minutes really familiarising yourself with the information.

Once you have an understanding of different treatments and their pros and cons, start by signing up to one online community (you can choose one from the Online Community Guide: http://simplifycancer.com/community/).

Five to 10 minutes a day is all it takes to get a feel for the type of questions that will come up in regards to your treatment, who the most active folks on the forum are, and how quickly people tend to respond.

PAINS AND ACHES DURING TREATMENT

Every time I have ever left things to chance, life has hit me square in the face. When I didn't stand up to the schoolyard bullies, the abuse only got worse. When I didn't speak up against a racist comment, I would just watch people continue to get away with them. When I didn't leave my ex even though I knew she cheated on me, I put up with the pain longer than was necessary.

Yes, drawing the cancer card from the deck of life is random, but our actions beyond the diagnosis need to be measured and deliberate.

When you combine the expertise of your medical team and the experience of cancer survivors, you start dealing with cancer on your own terms.

You know what's going on, you are in charge of the treatment process, and you prevent worry from running your life! It all starts with keeping track of your symptoms.

Before every checkpoint with your specialist, think: is there anything in particular that has been bothering you lately?

Anything in the weeks leading up to the appointment that you want to mention?

Anything odd or different, even if it seems unrelated?

The more uncomfortable you are about the thing that's bothering you, the more you need to get answers or it will only keep eating away at you, and that won't change until you know exactly what's going on and what you can do about it.

So take two minutes to think through your worries and write them down before your appointment.

Use a notepad or your phone.

Keeping track of your pains and aches becomes an important part of your process where you can **Integrate** your symptom into the treatment process:

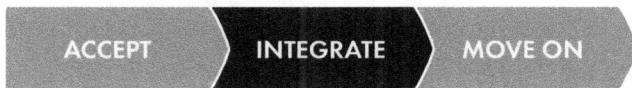
ACCEPT ▸ INTEGRATE ▸ MOVE ON

You can't be over prepared—no matter what, the more you know, the less you worry.

When you have a process for dealing with worries, you are in control of the situation.

You know what to do next and where to get answers; it becomes a natural part of your life during treatment.

Sometimes it's hard to imagine a different life waiting for you at the end of it, but it's there and you're going to get there!

You are going to get through it and one day look back on it as it becomes a distant memory.

But for now, you're going to make your way through cancer treatment and take your mind away from pain or stress.

Like a torch to light your way through the darkness, you want to have a singular reason that carries you through.

When I'm in pain or going through a tough situation, I find a moment that I treasure, a memory that drags me away from the reality that I'm facing:

As I make my way into the day oncology unit for my chemo infusion, I'm dreading the moment when I get the cannula in my arm.

My veins are tricky and it takes a few tries to get it right. I want to get my mind as far away as possible.

As I'm sitting in that chair with my arm out, I imagine myself back at home having a pillow fight with my son.

He's jumping on the bed, laughing, throwing the pillow at me. His laughter is infectious; the sunlight streams through the window.

By then, the drip is already in my vein.

Who is there in your life, waiting for you on the other side of cancer?

When you have a reason that touches you on a deep level, a reason that speaks to you and you alone in a powerful way, this reason changes your physiology.

It bypasses your pain censors, and lights you up when things are dark.

To anchor it in your mind, you want to find the right moment, and sometimes you need to clarify exactly what that looks like.

Who makes you happy? What does happiness look like to you?

Is it finishing school? Or getting a job? Becoming free of debt? Finding the person you love?

How would you know if you have achieved your goals?

What can you see in front of you?

What can you hear?

What does it feel like to touch?

This image may only be a few seconds long, but it is filled with enough emotion and detail that can bring it to life in an instant, and it's always sure to move you.

Hold it in your mind, see what it feels like, and if it feels right, if it rings true for you, then you know that it's authentic and real.

Now, what is the one word that is going to remind you about it? You can mentally hit the save button and store it. By associating a single word to this idea, you can draw it forth to your mind at any moment. This image that you hold on to does not even have to exist in the real world just yet; it can be a part of the future that you want to make true.

This is not daydreaming, but building the foundation for realizing your dreams.

For if you can't imagine it, how can it come true?

Is there is a bigger cause that hits home for you, like helping people you care about, or being a better person in the world in a way that is meaningful and personal to you?

When this cause is personal, when it's connected to something that has affected your life in a profound way, it's bound to drive you and make a difference for the sake of others.

And in acting on this drive, not only can you make a difference to other people who go through the same experiences, but it will change things for you too.

A powerful cause that speaks to you will take the attention away from cancer and towards making a real difference to a person who is struggling.

It can be something that you have experienced yourself, or something that touched you in some way.

You can take this cause and break it down to a moment in time.

Imagine you are speaking up against rape as a survivor— you're up on stage speaking about the horror of not knowing what to do and how you found a way of talking about it.

And there's a kid who's sitting in the very last row who's been hiding in misery and shame for years.

He's soaking in your every word, and it's a revelation—he's not alone anymore, he can speak up and tell his story and face the abuse he has suffered for years.

His revelation is the other side of your trauma.

So, what is on the other side of your cancer? Who matters most to you? Who can't you live without?

Finding internal reasons is very powerful. For example, when I wanted to give up smoking, I quit in a day because I saw what addiction had done to my friends.

It's not a mysterious superpower of the will—it's just a matter of finding a deep-rooted reason to make it through.

You just have to uncover your key reason for surviving cancer.

This reason, this powerful, singular vision can be the current that carries you through the treacherous waters of dark thoughts and confusion!

HOW TO DIFFERENTIATE BETWEEN CANCER, SIDE EFFECTS, AND UNRELATED PAIN

You may be going about your day just as you always do when an ache or pain sets you off.

In a different time, you might have paid it no mind.

But right now, you can't stop thinking about it—what if it's the cancer, or a side effect from treatment?

Or something else altogether?

What if it gets worse, or affects my treatment, or screws up my entire life?!

And what happens when I'm gone for good?

My friends—would they truly miss me?

Or hell, even remember me?

Would my wife find another man, a replacement?

These worrisome thoughts sneak up on you and take over everything you know and trust.

They can then spiral out of control, becoming more troublesome and irrational at every turn.

We want to take the raw emotion out of the situation and replace it with logic so that you can weigh things properly and decide what to do next. This is where you will use something I call the 4 Gates of Stability—a simple four-step process to work through your worries in a deliberate and methodical manner.

The first step is the Sanity check, where the purpose is to stop your mind from wandering off in any number of directions at a million miles an hour so that you can analyse the situation and work out a plan of action.

SANITY › SURVIVOR › SPECIALIST › SUPPORTER

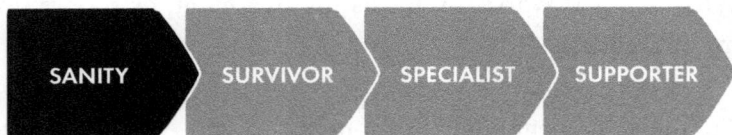

Make no assumptions before evidence—you want to examine what you are dealing with in a measured, rational way.

To get those worries out of your head, you are going to use a simple tool that I call an Outcome Map.

It enables you visualise all the possibilities of a situation so you can decide what to do next.

You will only need a pen, paper, and five minutes.

In the middle of the page, write down the specific pain, ache or other worry that's troubling you right now. Next, write down each probable outcome.

This could it be a side effect that you read about, a complication from treatment, muscle problem, or something else entirely.

When you have all the possibilities in front of you, spend 30 seconds on each one to think through how likely each outcome actually is.

It doesn't have to be perfect—we want to have all the likely scenarios written out to see.

Here is an example for a specific ache, pain, or worry:

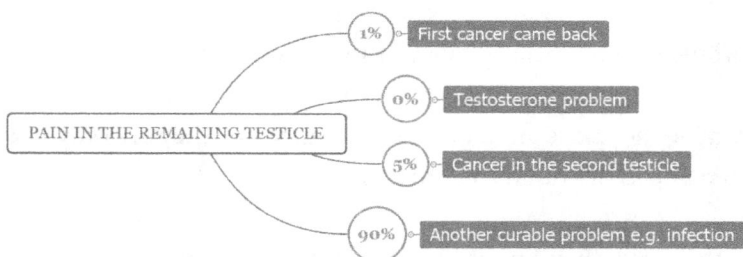

Now that it's all laid out in front of you, it's time to decide what the next best course of action is.

What is the one thing you can do about it today?

Is it serious enough to go to the hospital?

Will you call up your specialist?

Or see your family doctor?

For more examples and a video walkthrough of the Outcome Map, go here: http://canceroutcomemap.com

While your experience with cancer is unique, there are people who have been in the same situation as you are now.

They have been through your treatment and had to sort through their own pains and aches.

Wouldn't it be great to talk to those people about it?

Maybe they have already survived cancer, or they are only one step ahead of you in the process.

Either way, they know exactly what it's like and they understand the value of sharing that experience and supporting one another through tough times.

There are online communities around your type of cancer so you can get answers about things that are bothering you right now.

This is part two in our process: the Survivor check.

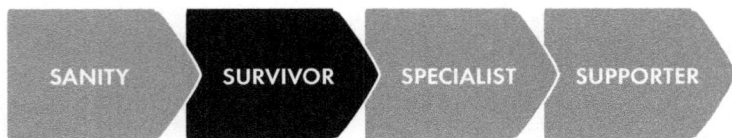

This is your direct line for getting the answers and support you need, all in a matter of hours.

The power lies in the fact that every person here knows exactly what you're going through, so they're eager to help.

There are no egos, no pressures, and no one knows who you are, so you don't even have to share your name; you only have to create a username and password to get in.

Now, it would be great to run into people like that on the street, but that can be hard to do depending on your circumstances, so the easiest thing to do is find them online!

To save you the time and hassle of finding the right one, I put together a free Online Community Guide that lists the top three online communities for most cancers: http://simplifycancer.com/community/

When you are posting your question, you want to make it easy for the person who is scanning the forum to decide if this is something they can help with.

Think of your topic title like a subject line for an email.

Its sole purpose is to help you decide whether you want to read the rest of the message or not.

Within hours, you will have some input and know whether it's something you need to worry about and what you can do right now.

The third step is your Specialist check, where your goal is to get timely advice from a medical expert.

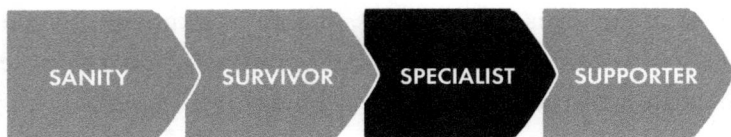

SANITY › SURVIVOR › **SPECIALIST** › SUPPORTER

Your specialist will always want to know how you are doing— or they should, if they are any good! If something is bothering you, don't wait until the next appointment—call the hospital or your specialist's office: "Hi, I am a patient of such and such and I have an urgent issue I need to speak to him/her about. Can I book a time to see him/her as soon as possible?"

If the first available appointment is too far away, ask for a callback.

If you don't hear back that day, find out if there is an oncology nurse you can reach out to.

If they aren't available either, next in line is your family doctor, whose primary role is triage, so if he or she can't answer your specific question, it's their job to find someone who can.

The fourth and most important step is your Supporter check.

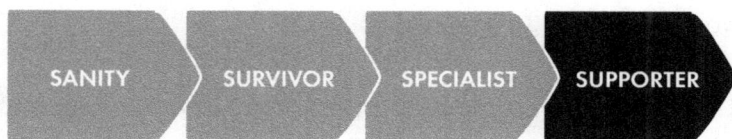

SANITY   SURVIVOR   SPECIALIST   SUPPORTER

It's great to be able handle some issues in life on your own.

Cancer is not one of them.

Now is the time to reach out to your people and let them know how they can be there for you.

Let's face it, if you are not going to get their support now, then you never will!

No one knows you like your partner or your close friend; they care about you, and they will always be there for you when you tell them what you need.

In a way, keeping worries to yourself is selfish because you keep your close friends in the dark, which makes it harder for them to feel connected and needed in your life. The people who care about you genuinely want to help you, even if just in some small way. If you tell them what you want them to do and include them in the process, both of you will benefit and grow your relationship.

At any stage, talk to someone you trust—your partner, relative, a friend. If you don't have anyone that you want to share your worries with, find a professional.

There are fantastic counsellors, psychologists. and help line operators out there who specifically work with people like you and me, people who go through cancer.

They won't judge you—they know how to listen and they want to help.

Following these four steps will help you deal with worries that come up during treatment in a much healthier and more productive way.

Having a process puts you in control of the situation because you can assess your symptoms in a calm, rational way.

Which brings us to **Move On**, the third step of AIM in relation to treatment.

When you build trust with your medical team and build a better understanding of how to deal with treatment, you can move on with your life despite cancer.

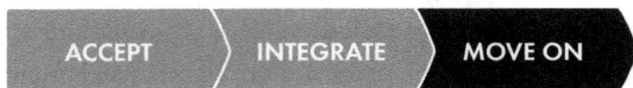

ACCEPT INTEGRATE MOVE ON

WRAP-UP AND ACTION STEPS

Use the checklist below to decide what actions you are going to take for restoring calm and control during your cancer treatment:

✔ To help me make decisions about treatment, I will set up a follow up appointment with my specialist at the end of our meeting.

✔ To help me make decisions about treatment, I will get a second opinion with another specialist by asking my doctor for the referral.

✔ I will ask my oncologist / nurse / specialist / _____ for their email / phone number / best method of contact.

_____

_____

_____

✔ I like the idea of having a designated worry time and I have scheduled mine to happen at _____ _____.

_____

_____

_____

✔ I will break my worries apart by writing them down every _____.

_____

_____

_____

_____

✔ I will use an Outcome Map for specific worries.

_____

_____

_____

_____

✔ I will get rid of worry through exercise and physical
movement by _____
every _____.

_____

_____

_____

_____

When you are prepared and take meaningful action,
you know what's coming your way and how to deal
with it.

My hope is that some of these actions make sense to
where you are right now and that you are ready to make
it happen in your life to get through treatment and have
the life you want despite cancer.

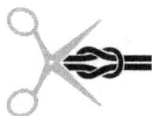

WHO IS GOING TO BE THERE FOR ME?

FLYING IN THE FACE OF DANGER

It's a tough, upward climb through cancer, and it's even harder to do it alone.

Where do you find the strength to deal with the stress and the madness of it all?

You don't have an infinite supply of strength available to you, so how do you get more of it when your energy's run out?

This strength has to come from somewhere, and I believe that the source is the people in your life—people who don't get in the way, who are not showy or superficial, who want to be there for you and support you on your terms rather than bringing their own agendas into your treatment.

Most of us are lucky to have those people with us, and yet, we often leave them on the sidelines at the times when we need each other the most.

Even worse, we often don't give them a chance to step up and be there for us in a real, meaningful way!

For example, imagine you're on a plane. It's a flight which you've done a million times before.

You are in your seat, flicking through a magazine to pass the time.

Suddenly, the plane starts to shake, emergency lights flicker, an alarm goes off on the loudspeakers.

Someone is screaming at the top of their lungs as you try to put your life mask on.

The plane takes a nosedive and panic sets in—everyone is freaking out and you are trying to put on your life jacket.

It all becomes a blur—there's an impact, you scramble out of the wreckage, and now you're in the water trying to catch your breath.

At this moment, would it be okay to ask for help?

Yes, of course; your life is on the line and you need all the help and support you can get. This seems obvious, right?

So why is it that we don't feel like asking for help is okay when we crash into cancer?

Cancer does not have the immediacy of a plane crash, but it's a life-threatening situation all the same.

You are trying to stay afloat when things get out of control and you don't want your family and friends to freak out, or worse, feel sorry for you or go out of their way to support you, yet you need them to be there for you on your side.

After all, this is cancer, and it is going to be tough, but it gets easier when you bring your people into your corner.

The support from your people is not a switch that can be flicked on and off.

It's a chain process that you begin with a charge.

Your charge, your energy is what draws your people together to light up the room!

This energy is what drives you onward as you go through treatment; it is what pulls you through when you're in pain, and what lifts you up when you're stuck in limbo, waiting for your next scan result!

It's the backing you get from your partner, your family, your friends, your medical team, the people around you.

But in order for them to be there for you, you've got to let them in and be open and direct about what is bothering you right now.

Because your true supporters want the real story. It's only natural to **Accept** that you should never deal with cancer on your own!

This is the first step towards getting your supporters to be there for you in a real, meaningful way:

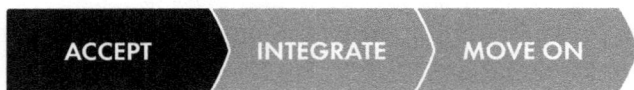

ACCEPT › INTEGRATE › MOVE ON

When you talk about your worries, there is no need for drama, no need for epic revelations or teary-eyed confessions.

You're having an authentic conversation about things that are important to you right now.

And it's such a relief when you don't have to overthink your conversations, when you're open and direct about where you're at.

One of the ways I've transitioned into opening up has been by no longer saying "I'm fine" when people ask me how I'm going.

In the long run it has been so much easier to blurt out something that's been eating away at me for days:

> *"I've got this test coming up next week, that's when I'm going to find out if the treatment has worked or not, and I'm freaking out, because it can change my life in a big way."*

When you lay it all out, there are no awkward moments, and your people don't have to guess what's on your mind.

Because you can always tell when the person is brooding over something, especially when it's your partner or a close friend.

There are little signs that you can't even put into words, and you don't want to ask about it directly because you could be wrong and you don't want to make things worse.

The unspoken worry hangs heavy in the air and it puts everyone on edge, dragging you down even further.

But when you can casually bring your worries out into the open, it makes the whole interaction flowing and natural.

Your conversation becomes more authentic and real because you're not thinking about what you should and should not say. You have nothing to hide when you don't attempt to protect those you care about from worry.

They can take on a lot more than you think when they know what you are dealing with. Opening up doesn't have to be anything epic or sophisticated, you're just being honest and direct about things that are bothering you right now.

Of course, it doesn't mean you're going to talk about cancer all the time—that would drive you crazy!

Most of the time, you just want to talk about things that have nothing to do with cancer, and you would only bring it up when it's something specific that's troubling you right now.

And when you do talk about your worries, they lose their grip on you.

When you give your worries away, their gravity deflates.

You now have a lot more room for things you care about!

'Support' smacks of grand gestures, of being superficial and fake, but really, it's the little things that can lift you up:

- Hearing a friendly voice when you are you are feeling like junk during treatment
- Sharing a joke to break up the agonising wait for your test results
- Dropping by with a meal when you can't be bothered cooking
- Driving you to the hospital so you can talk about anything other than cancer

True support, like friendship, is never planned; it springs up on its own, often when you least expect it.

True support is mutual; you are there for each other when times get tough.

Don't turn your people away—let them know how they can be there for you!

HOW TO GET THE SUPPORT YOU WANT FROM PEOPLE IN YOUR LIFE

It's so easy to get caught off guard when something throws you off.

Let's say you are walking down the street.

It's a nice day and you are enjoying the time alone with your thoughts when a car speeds past you; with an agonising screech it slams into a tree…

So, what do you do now?

Do you call the ambulance, or the police?

Or do you jump in and help the driver out of the wreckage?

Is that even safe? Could your help inadvertently do more damage? Should you leave it to the authorities and stay out of the way?

And there are other people around—surely, someone has already called for help…

It's easy to lose yourself in a moment when you are face to face with an unexpected turn of events.

This is the reality many of your friends and family find themselves in when they find out you have cancer.

They want to help, they want to be there for you, but they don't know how.

They don't want to say or do the wrong thing because they don't want to look stupid or insensitive, or make you feel worse.

Often, they end up taking an easier route—doing nothing.

This is the time for you to guide them in how to do the right thing by you.

Give them a chance to step up and prove themselves as your true supporters!

The best way to do that is by explicitly telling them about the help you are looking for.

This will eliminate guesswork and misunderstanding because you make it clear what you expect to happen.

You don't need to do it face to face—you can make a list of things you want help with and email it to your people.

Unlike social media, email lets you speak directly to specific people, and only them.

Put together an email that spells out exactly what you want, without being dramatic or needy.

Here is the email that I would write, if I had to do it all over again:

Hi all,

As you may or may not know, I was recently diagnosed with _____ *cancer.*

If you want to know how the treatment works, here is a quick overview:

On dd/mm/yyyy, I will be starting _____ *(chemo, procedure, radiation).*

I have no idea how things will turn out, but feel free to ask me anything. You can also visit me in the hospital—I will be staying at _____ *between* _____ *and* _____.

The whole thing really sucks and we're in for a rough ride so I'd really appreciate your help with any of this:

1. Getting to and from the hospital
2. Getting groceries (once a week)
3. Babysitting

If there's something you'd like to volunteer for, let me know.

Thanks,
Joe

I've put together three more email templates for you here: http://simplifycancer.com/scbookbundle

No guesswork, no misunderstanding, no excuses.

That's how you **Integrate** your experience into your support system—making your cancer worries a part of the conversation:

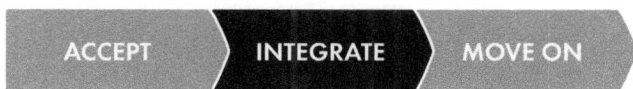

ACCEPT · INTEGRATE · MOVE ON

When you get your people to help you in a meaningful way, your true supporters are going to be grateful because you just made it easy for them to be there for you, without being needy or weird.

They don't need to pretend like they care—they will prove it to you beyond any doubt by supporting you in the way that you want to be supported. Then, you can take charge of the situation in a way that is going to give you the strength you need to deal with cancer.

3 REASONS WHY SOME PEOPLE TURN AWAY FROM YOU DURING CANCER

With chemo, the unreality of the situation had me cornered.

This cancer, this treatment, none of it seemed right, it was never supposed to happen...

Not to me, anyhow. You always think that cancer is something that only happens to other people.

And that's what's scary about getting diagnosed; when all bets are off, you have no idea how this treatment is going to work out.

If only this treatment came with a guarantee signed by the oncologist, a promise that it was definitely going to work...

I would frame it up on the wall as a reminder that everything was going to turn out just fine! But nothing is for certain anymore, you are hoping against hope now.

I needed strength to get through, some reminder that I didn't dream it all up, the drip in my hand, the hospital visits... Then I realised—my friends, they would lend me their strength to get through this treatment and beyond. Using technology to band us together, reaching out to me has never been easier, and yet...

There were no phone calls, no messages, no emails.

"What is happening?" I thought.

This couldn't be right—these are my closest friends, after all!

There had to be a problem, some kind of glitch in the network.

Or maybe the reception was jammed at the hospital due to all the equipment.

Yes, that must be it!

To confirm my theory, I stumbled out into the ward to find a landline. I dialled my mobile expecting voicemails, only to have the phone light up, playing a silly jingle again.

For several long seconds, I stared at it, transfixed, refusing to accept my new reality.

And then it hit me…

Nobody was coming.

The people I trusted, the people I thought I knew, they chose to abandon me at the time when I needed them most.

And it was a choice, conscious or otherwise.

In a matter of weeks, the way I saw myself had unravelled in the most spectacular fashion.

And it hurt worse than the pain I was in. At least with cancer it's nothing personal...

Months later, after working through this and cross checking with fellow cancer travellers, I found out that this is to be expected.

It happens to most of us—there is always at least one person who is not where you want them to be, and it comes down to these three reasons:

1. They are awkward about death and dying, and you having cancer gets in the way of supporting you.

2. They are afraid of looking stupid and insensitive by saying the wrong thing. They don't want to feel judged and they don't want to lose face if they can help it.
   Often, this is the person who genuinely wants to be there for you but doesn't know how. They need your guidance to support you on your terms, so let them know—give them a chance to step up and be there for you!

3. Sometimes, you grow distant with people.
   Because it happens over time, you don't notice it, not at first.

And it can take something like cancer to bring this to light and make you see things in a different way.

It hurts when they have no room for you in their life, but there is nothing you can do to change it.

Except doing the right thing for yourself—putting your energy towards those people who stand by your side as you go through cancer, who support you on your terms.

With cancer, the true nature of things is revealed.

It may not be what you want or expect, but it is what is real.

Finally, you can **Move On** with your life towards people that are there for you, people who listen and pay attention, who put you ahead of their own issues:

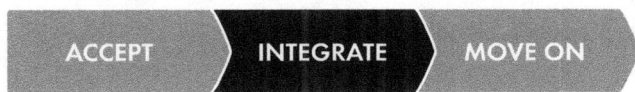

ACCEPT INTEGRATE MOVE ON

Cancer helped me to start judging people in my life by what they do, not what they say.

Those who are there for you, they aren't doing it to tick a box or make a show of it.

They just show up.

So when an old friend came to visit me at the hospital, I knew that she came to be by my side and listen.

And it was such a relief to be heard—nothing else mattered.

There was no need to put on a brave face because I wasn't judged on my performance, and I could speak my mind freely.

And it felt right, to be myself, to be honest and direct, without any drama or show, to bask in her full and undivided attention, and to march my worries out and far away. It's important to find those who truly listen—especially if you are prone to keeping to yourself and letting things build up inside of you—because ultimately, you want a way to let it go so that you can move on with your life during treatment.

Yes, some people are going to fall short of where you want them to be, but there will be plenty who will stand by you through cancer, on your terms.

Being open and transparent about what you want and what you need is the best way to weed out the pretenders so that you can focus on those who care about you.

Embrace your true supporters, and give the rest a chance to get out of your way.

LOOKING OUT FOR YOUR TRUE SUPPORTERS

Before starting chemo, I took my three year old son to our favourite park.

It had a little pond, and a playground, and it's very quiet, especially on a weekday.

I couldn't stop laughing as Michael chased the seagulls, and we had sandwiches and sultanas under a palm tree.

It was a perfect day, a day I wanted to last forever... So when the treatment began, I didn't want to frighten him, so the message to him was—daddy is sick, and the doctors are dealing with it.

But when I looked at Michael as he was sitting on my hospital bed, I saw the hurt in his eyes.

It was the hurt of not being privy to some hidden knowledge, a secret not shared between us.

That's when I realised that by wanting to shield my boy from my cancer, I had excluded him.

This is what ultimately creates suffering for you and those who care about you.

It saps away the strength and resilience to deal with treatment and life beyond.

And those unsaid words are instruments of torture for people you love.

Because your loved ones are hit the hardest.

Your mother, your partner, your closest friend.

Their entire worlds turn inside out. They can't bear a future without you in it.

It's cruel and terrifying to watch you suffer while still having to deal with their everyday life, which doesn't stop even when their loved one is going through cancer…

Their thoughts are now occupied by fear for you, for your life, for what you have together.

The future, once clear, is now obscured by the unknown.

And it seems like there is nothing they can do to change things, to make you feel better…

But you can change that!

You can tell them straight up about what you are going through and how they can help.

Do you want to be around people?

Do you need alone time?

Is there something you want to do more of?

You know what's good for you, but your closest allies, your unconditionals, they can't read your mind—you've got to tell them about what you are going through!

They can take it.

Whatever it is for you, don't lock yourself away and keep them guessing!

There is no need to "take it like a man," to march on as if everything is just fine.

This is cancer, you don't need to put on a brave face!

The manly thing is to put your closest allies first and give them the comfort of being there for you, on your terms.

Tell them exactly what you need—and if that means asking them to give you headspace, so be it.

We expect others to intuitively figure out what we want, but for those who haven't had the direct experience of dealing with cancer, the reality isn't so clear and the proper response is elusive.

But nothing is worse than silence.

It has the power of breaking the strongest bonds.

Our ability to read others gets a knock under duress, so speaking out is more vital than ever.

The worst thing you can do is to try and suffocate your fear by keeping it to yourself.

It will only build up, slowly, until it breaks out to put you in a panic and take it out on people you care about—maybe it's your lover, your mother, or a friend.

It's never simple to put this into practice when you are on the edge, but think—can you find a way to include others without conflicts or old habits getting in the way?

Is there something you can do together that you would all enjoy, or that would at least allow you to get along?

Maybe going to a see a sports game, or out for a coffee, or home for dinner.

Talk about it to as many people as possible—your partner, family, work mates.

Yes, it's awkward and often comes out the wrong way, but none of this is your fault.

If they ask you how you're going, tell them what's going on for you right now—there's no reason to keep it to yourself!

And there is no need for drama—just blurt out whatever is on your mind when they ask. When you instruct your people on how they can help you, they are going to step up and respond in a powerful way by taking meaningful action because they know exactly what you expect from them now.

Taking a moment to say thanks goes a long way to show it means a lot to you and that you don't take it for granted.

Support from people you care about is only going to pull you up instead of further drag you down with worries and uncertainty.

Accept that you can't and shouldn't do it on your own, and that the best thing you can do for yourself is to guide your people to how they can be there for you.

Integrate their support into your everyday life by making it a part of the conversation.

When you appreciate those who are there for you, you are also giving a chance for the remaining few to step back so you can **Move On** with your life.

WRAP-UP AND ACTION STEPS

Look at things through the eyes of your loved ones—what's it like for them right now?

Ask yourself:

Do they know what's on my mind?

Am I being self-centred, dismissive, or harsh?

Use these statements as your action steps for your true supporters:

✔ I will talk about cancer to my family, including

_____.

✔ I am going to tell my family exactly how they can help me and not get in the way.

✔ Every day I am going to share with my partner what bothers me.

✔ I am going to tell my people how they can help via email.

✔ I am going to tell my people how they can help in person.

✔ I will explain my situation to people I work with and keep them informed.

✔ I will provide advice and ways around situations for people I work with while I'm dealing with cancer.

✔ I will ring my cancer non-profit to ask about legal, financial, medical, and other services they have that can help me right now.

_____

_____

_____

_____

✔ I will keep my people informed about my cancer through _____
(email, social media, in person meetings)

_____

_____

_____

✔ I will allow myself to rant about cancer to a few people in my life, including _____.

_____

_____

_____

✔ I will talk to a person outside of my social circle who doesn't know me and has no agenda.

When your world is under attack, you bring your supporters on your side by making them a part of your world where you are dealing with cancer.

People who care will thank you for being frank and honest, so don't leave them guessing where your head is at and how they can be there for you.

This is a real man's true superpower—putting those close to you first, and your ego off to the side.

And you know what?

In the midst of all the craziness, it's easy to forget the little things:

A thank you, a kind word, a smile.

These tokens of gratitude create enormous goodwill and positivity to help you and your loved ones through treatment.

It seems obvious, but we don't do it enough!

Pain and worries, they get to you, and it's so easy to let those simple things slip, to take the people you care about for granted.

With cancer, empty words mean nothing—this is where good intentions go to die.

The authentic is separated from the false, once and forever more.

Embrace those whose words of support are backed up by their actions—you have no time or energy to spare for the rest.

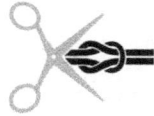

HOW DO I DEAL WITH WAITING AND UNCERTAINTY?

HOW TO DIVERT YOUR THOUGHTS AWAY FROM CANCER

Here is the one thing that cancer-free people can never understand...

This cancer you have is not a broken leg that makes it a little awkward to get around.

It takes over what's inside, it plays games with your mind.

These worrisome thoughts are never far away, lurking around in the shadows, just waiting for the right moment to pounce...

Even when you're talking with your loved one, or picking out groceries, you're thinking about how much time you still have, or what happens when you die, and wondering what the point of it all is…

You try to swat those thoughts away:

> *"I don't want to think about it, damn it, go away and leave me alone!"*

Yet it only makes things worse.

I found a way to divert these thoughts away from cancer, at a time when I least expected it…

It was on a regular walk during treatment—walking was a way to check for lung damage during chemo.

To be honest, it wasn't much fun.

Each night, I stumbled along the railway tracks like a zombie, ears ringing, mind wading about in a fog, my hands and legs trying to catch up with the body.

My thoughts were muted, a potent cocktail of confusion and fear.

The chemo drugs drained my energy like a vampire.

Slow and deliberate, I would force myself to take another step.

Forward!

Away from the pain that was taking over the body and the worry that was taking over the mind.

"Enough! I'm done with having my entire life on pause, constantly waiting to be told what's next.

Cancer is a part of my life for now, and I can't run away anymore.

I can't have my life here on this side and have cancer over on the other side.

These two lives don't run parallel—I can't think about two different things at the same time.

Two roads must merge into one.

One life, one direction, and then the road is clear."

In that instant, I found new colors in the world.

Bright, sprawling textures, pierced by the fading sunlight.

Everything has a purpose—the railway track in the ravine, the abandoned backyards, the chemicals in my blood, and they come together to create what I crave most of all…

This is freedom.

Freedom from living in the shadow of this disease.

Freedom to be with people I can't live without, to be myself, to live the life that made me happy.

That's when I came to terms with the reality of cancer. It's true, I can't change if this treatment is going to work or not, but that is the only thing that you can't influence.

So, what are all the things within your control?

First, how much you know about your treatment. When you put your trust in your medical team, you have complete confidence that all of your questions will be answered and how to find your specialist or nurse when you need to.

You can always book a follow-up appointment to clear things up, or have a phone number ready to ring to get your urgent questions answered.

When you understand how your treatment works and what it's all about, you are asking the necessary questions that allow you to make decisions about what's right for you and your life when it comes to treatment and life beyond cancer.

The second thing you can control is how to deal with obstacles that come up during and after treatment.

You never asked for this experience, but now that you are here, it helps to talk to people who have been through this before, who can give you advice on tackling a specific problem, be it a side effect from treatment, after effects, or pain, and share what they would do differently if given the chance.

You can find cancer survivors for your type of cancer using my free Online Community Guide: http://simplifycancer.com/community/

The type of support that you receive from people around you is entirely within your control—truth is, most people want to be there for you, but they don't know how, so it's your responsibility to be explicit about what's going on with you and how they can help.

You can do this without drama, just being honest and direct about what's happening when they ask you about how you're doing, or when something is bothering you.

Remember that you can also talk to the people you work with about your cancer and how they can support you. This way, you're giving yourself the headspace you need to concentrate on getting through treatment, work part-time through recovery, or leave early to get to your specialist appointment.

Life doesn't stop when you get cancer, and you have the power to put things in motion to make things easier along the way.

Most of us don't want advice from people we don't know, but then again, most of us are not dealing with a life-threatening situation like cancer where a different perspective can make a huge difference to how you get through it.

So talking to your hospital and your cancer non-profit about legal and financial help is so crucial—they will share things that will make your life easier.

There are so many great services that you might have never taken advantage of because you didn't know they were there for you.

I only found out about many of these services through talking to people on my podcast when I no longer needed services that are there for you throughout treatment.

And that's a shame, because it would have been a great help!

An oncology nurse hotline that can answer questions about treatment, an exercise physiologist who can set up a personalized exercise routine to speed up your recovery after treatment, a licensed dietitian who can help you find the right foods to get you through treatment, financial support during treatment, a qualified counsellor or psychologist who can give you advice on dealing with stress and tension throughout cancer—these are just some of the many lesser known options available to you.

I'm sure that some of these services, like talking to a counsellor, are outside the norm for you—I know that was the case for me, but this situation that you are in right now with cancer is far from normal too.

No one is there to judge you, and these are the tools that can help you along the way and make things easier. Give them a try! It will give you the freedom from worrying about what else can go wrong when there is so much to make right.

After all, hope is the only thing stronger than fear.

When you shift your thoughts away from uncertainty and towards things you can influence or control, you give yourself the freedom to deal with cancer on your terms.

HOW TO COMBAT THE PARALYSING WAIT FOR RESULTS

With cancer, you're constantly waiting for something to happen—the next appointment, the next treatment session, the next test result...

It's hard when you're caught up in this new state of a constant in between, when everything hinges on a new piece of information or diagnosis.

Thoughts are slippery, the mind longs for any certainty it can find, something to cling to for a while. Sometimes I hate myself for it—for not being able to think straight, for not pulling myself together when I want to, for falling down the spiral of doom and paranoia from just one tiny thought.

It may only be a half-formed suggestion, a tiny whisper of doubt, but this worry, it takes root in your mind and grows, until eventually you lose the thread of what started it and you are left with paralyzing fear and hopelessness...

How do you keep your balance when everything in your life has become fluid and uncertain?

To drive that uncertainty back and prevent your worries from taking over, you need an anchor to tie you to the reality of what is happening so that you can rationally think about where you are right now.

We can apply our Outcome Map to stay on top of worries and uncertainty, to ground you in the facts of what you are dealing with right now and stop your imagination from going out of control.

If you remember from earlier in the book, the Outcome Map is a tool to help you visualise all the possibilities of a situation so you can put it into perspective and decide what to do next, free of irrational worry.

You will only need five minutes for this.

Take out a piece of paper and write down your next milestone (your first post treatment checkup, for example).

Then, write out each possible outcome (cancer has gone, tumor has shrunk, it's grown, no change), the likelihood of each outcome as a percentage, and what you will need to do in each case.

Now you can look at it objectively and decide what you can do about it today.

Take this map with you, whether it's on a piece of paper or you've taken a photo of it to keep on your phone, so that when you start to worry, you can pull it up and re-orientate yourself around what is going on and stop irrational thoughts and uncertainty from pulling you aside.

Here is an example from my life before my first checkup post treatment.

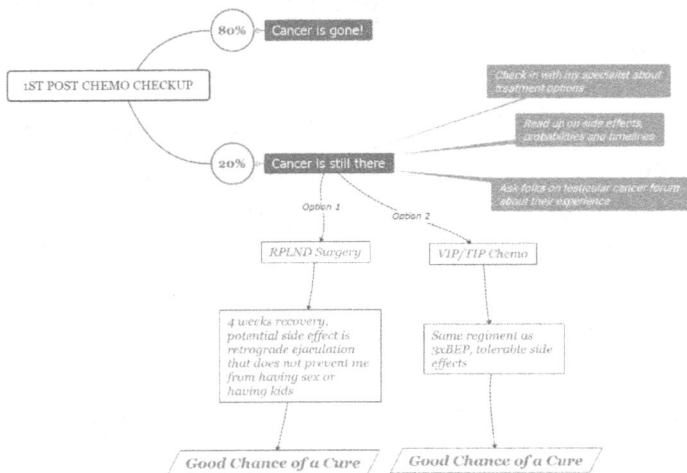

Having worked through your worries methodically, you are safe with the knowledge that you did everything in your power to be ready for it, and the rest is out of your hands.

And when it gets to you, you can honestly say to yourself, "I'll worry about it later."

Whenever you set aside time for worrying if the cancer is spreading or if the treatment has worked, time yourself with a stopwatch on your phone.

Take the worry that's spinning around in your mind, put it in the spotlight, and turn it this way and that in your mind.

Ask yourself:

Is the worry real?

What are the chances that it's going to come true?

Can you do anything about it? Can you ask your specialist, talk to your doctor, or check in with your cancer community online? Can you talk it through with your partner or a friend to see if you are overreacting, or to just vent?

Choose one thing that you're going to do about it today; when you take immediate action, you are in control of the situation.

POISE: 1ˢᵀ SUPPORT PILLAR TO RESTORE STABILITY AND CALM

Like overflowing storm water, worrisome thoughts can take over and destroy your balance and control.

We can't stop these thoughts from coming on naturally, but we can channel these thoughts away to a place where it's not running your life.

To divert these thoughts, I have three ideas that can help you right now.

These are the 3 Support Pillars for you to lean on during the times of stress and uncertainty throughout cancer.

On the first day of chemo, as the liquid from the black bag slowly descended into my vein, I thought of my son—how would he remember me?

Or rather, how did I want him to remember me? As someone strong and courageous?

Always looking on the bright side of life?

Or maybe, as someone who makes decisions, who is always in control of the situation?

None of it rang true, until I stumbled on one word—fun.

I want him to remember the fun times we'd had together: the pillow fights, new adventures every weekend, lazing about on the couch, chasing each other around in the backyard…

That's it! I knew I struck gold, and fun became my motto.

Whenever we were home, a light would go off in my head—fun, that's what we want now! I'd tickle him, chase him around the house, or make up some silly song about a dolphin and a dragon being friends.

Within a week, I saw a profound change in him—yes, he expected his silly daddy to goof around, but on a deeper level, what was going to stand out for him in the years to come were the carefree days of his childhood.

What's more, I began to feel more comfortable with myself and our way of life.

I no longer felt guilty about giving him ice cream before dinner and I didn't beat myself up over not teaching him to ride a bike.

I then started to apply this mindset to how I was with my wife and my mum by choosing one overarching quality that I wanted to get across, and over time, they too responded in a powerful way.

This gave me a certain poise, a higher level of carrying myself because it gave me so much more comfort with my vision of myself as opposed to beating myself up over how I should be.

It made me calmer and more collected, because when you're focused, when you are fully present, then you're just in it, you're not worried about cancer or what might happen next. This is the way things are meant to be—a natural outcome of your relationship, with no conscious effort involved on your part.

This process, which I call **Selective Memory** has changed my relationships and my vision of myself for the better, and it can do the same for you and your life!

When you think about the three people you care about the most, how do you want them to see you?

Write down the person's name and find one word that sums up this quality.

This keyword then becomes a trigger for you to show the side of yourself that you want to shine the most around them.

It's the living, breathing legacy that is created in every moment—every time you are around your child, your partner, your best friend—so that when they think of you, they get the best version of you, the one you dedicate to them!

At first, you remind yourself every time you are around them by thinking of your keyword, but within days, it becomes second nature. Eventually it is nothing more than a logical extension of your relationship without any conscious effort involved on your part.

This feeling takes center stage to forge an ever-strengthening bond.

You are completely immersed in the moment, and that's when you create the ultimate poise that brings more balance into your life.

PLACEMENT: 2ND SUPPORT PILLAR TO RESTORE STABILITY AND CALM

While you can't stop worrying about pain or the next checkup, you can get on top of the tension and stress that builds up in your body.

But how do you do that?

It was on my mind for the longest time until I decided to try out every de-stressing approach I could think of—from mindfulness to meditation and yoga…

None of these approaches worked.

In a weird way, I felt completely relaxed as I was lying on the floor with my eyes closed or twisting myself into a pretzel, but it did not take away the underlying tension and worry that I was experiencing day to day. So, what was wrong?

What I discovered with a lot of trial and error was that relief from stress and tension comes through intense focus, not relaxation.

In the past, we were told that rest is the remedy for every ailment, yet we now know that it's not always the case.

You release this energy through movement when you consistently push yourself forward.

Research tells us that exercise is not only a powerful tool for circumventing stress, but it also helps with treatment-related fatigue, like "chemo brain" and other side effects that come with cancer.

I love running and resistance training because I can do it on my own and it's easy to plan around, but many folks who went through cancer prefer cycling, football, or surfing.

Ultimately, it's important to choose what's right for you—something that you can keep doing without forcing yourself through it.

Exercise physiologists can help you by tailoring an exercise program for you so that you're consistently pushing yourself just enough to get results (have more energy, clear your head, lose weight), but not to the point where you're straining or harming yourself in the process.

For mental focus, the best exercise that I can recommend to you is chess because you have to constantly assess and take control of the situation. In order to figure out an opponent's strategy, you have to put yourself in their shoes and implement a plan to win.

You can't escape your worries during cancer—but you can release all that pent-up energy when you channel it towards physical and mental sports.

PURPOSE: 3ᴿᴰ SUPPORT PILLAR TO RESTORE STABILITY AND CALM

With cancer, it's so hard to make sense of everything that's happening.

I often find myself staring into space, thoughts jumbled together like spaghetti. There is no energy, no spark...

It can be hard to pick yourself up and get on with your daily life.

So one time, I thought to myself—if this was my last day, what would I do right now?

If there was no more time left, what could I still do today?

Immediately, I knew I had to be with my wife and my son, to soak in every moment, and to show my love in the simplest and most brutal way that I know—just being there, fully in the moment, without any distractions.

With the time I have, I want to leave a legacy of making a difference, helping people who need it, now and into the future, and that means working on my book.

I am going to have to wait for my test results, and that is out of my control, but that's the only thing that I'm willing to wait around for.

So how can I put off anything important in this life anymore?

When I ask myself what I would do if this was my last day alive, it clears up my priorities in an instant.

It even helps in the most mundane moments, like when I'm driving to work—I can't do anything about the traffic, so why get angry about something out of my control that I'll forget about the moment I'm out of it? I can use the time to do things I enjoy, like getting lost in the music I love or listening to the podcasts that I love.

In an instant, an incredible weight is lifted off my shoulders:

When I'm in a traffic jam, and there are cars cutting in in front of me, and I'm running late to pick up my kid from childcare, and I'm powerless to do anything about it, I ask myself—what if this was my last day in this life? What would I do?

Would I get angry? Would I wind myself up about it all?

No, I can only do my best, and so I put on the music that I love, and I think of the quiet night at home when I'm going to sit down with a good book and a stout, and that instantly puts me in a good place.

With this clarifying question, I no longer worry about the long list of things that need to be done at work, I can concentrate on the things that need to be done first. I don't do any over-time, I stay out of politics and drama, and I avoid egos and conflicts as best I can.

I stopped doing things out of habit when my heart was not in it, no longer following other people's agendas, and this cleared away commitments and expectations that I refuse to subscribe to.

My purpose is clear—and that has created the headspace that I need to focus on things that really matter to me, because everything else is a distraction.

The best thing is, meaningful plans make themselves now—it's a matter of natural selection.

I initially began prompting myself throughout the day, and it has gradually become a new, simpler way of life.

It's an incredible relief as it clears away those needless commitments that you sign up for, or other people's agendas, going through the motions when your heart is not in it, or when you're doing things out of habit alone.

Instead, you create more time to do the things that you care about.

It will allow you to reclaim the peace of mind that you need right now because you are bringing purpose to everything that you do!

And you already know your purpose—only you may not have spoken it out loud just yet.

Is there something you never got around to doing because you told yourself you never had the time?

What are you proud of on a deep, personal level that you can share with others to better their lives?

Did you struggle in your life in one way or another, and then found a way out?

Could it be that you are not giving yourself the credit for something that you are already doing right now?

It's all about being part of something that's bigger than you— that is going to be your legacy in the world. Something that has the power to make you happy and fulfilled because it aligns with your core values.

It's your personal mission to right the wrongs you see around you and do something about it, something that feels right on the inside.

You choose who you want to help, when, and how.

With clear and direct purpose in my life, every checkup and every medical scan is a checkpoint when I ask myself—have I been living my best life?

And if the answer is yes, then I know that no matter what happens, I don't have a single regret to live with.

ANY DAY, THIS CAN BE TAKEN AWAY

The warmth of her naked body presses against mine.

I don't want to wake her.

The warmth of her skin is a delicate drug. Its intensity is both overwhelming and soothing.

How can every tiny wrinkle add up to perfection?

One thought lingers: "Any day this can be taken away."

I smile, every second a privilege.

Time seems to stretch to infinity, but I know it's just a trick of the mind.

This is my life.

Mine. I don't ever want it to stop and I will never give it away.

I promise that no moment will be taken for granted, or forgotten about, or passed by, because any day it can be taken away—with or without cancer.

This is my mantra, an instant hit of right now, the only force that matters.

Experiencing the world the way a child does.

The future is distant and immense, the past insignificant and easily forgotten, with only the present to live for.

It's the blood running through your veins, the beat of your pulse—once you find it, you never let it go.

Can you feel it?

OUTRO

MY GRANDFATHER NEVER SPOKE OF the Holocaust. Not of the murders of his parents and two of his brothers; of every friend, foe, and familiar he had ever known; or of the war and how he got his limp.

But it could not break him.

He built his life along those memories and values most sacred, not the atrocities and horrors that haunted him.

Not ignore it, but live in spite of events that are beyond our control.

He learned how to heal.

How to fall in love, make a family, and save lives.

He chose to define himself by the memories he wanted to keep and share, and to grow the future he wanted to be a part of, no matter how scary the present was.

How is cancer going to define you, now that it's here? That is the choice only you can make.

You choose between the inevitable pain of treatment and the avoidable suffering that comes with keeping it all to yourself.

You choose a lonely misery or sharing your pain with your true supporters who want you to win.

You choose between worrying yourself sick or seeking out answers from the folks who went on this path before, who know what it's like and want to help you.

You have a choice: to curse your rotten luck, fate, and the mighty circumstance…

Or admit to what you always knew, but were never forced to confront—that life is unpredictable, precious, and worth its weight in gold.

That the only people who matter are the ones you can't be without.

That the only ambition worth pursuing is the one you want to be remembered for.

That the only lasting difference you make is for the people you care about.

That the only thing worth planning for is today, because cancer or not, you will never get it back.

But I want you to know that you are never alone!

I'm here for you.

Let me know how you are going, here is my email: joe@simplifycancer.com

And do check out the free gift bundle that I created just for you!

It includes the Simplify Cancer video course where I walk you through the key strategies in overcoming the four key challenges us men face during cancer, as well as the audiobook version that you can listen to when you're on the go or resting from treatment, and every actionable tool discussed in the book are now available absolutely free of charge.

Grab it here: http://simplifycancer.com/scbookbundle

It's a tough time, but you can do this, my friend, you can get through treatment and have the life that you truly deserve, despite cancer!

www.ingramcontent.com/pod-product-compliance
Lightning Source LLC
Chambersburg PA
CBHW021830020426
42334CB00014B/561